Get Fit Anywhere

Twelve weeks to a leaner, stronger body

By

Stephen Robson

Contents

Introduction

Basic nutrition

The plan

Workout 1 Exercises

Workout 2 Exercises

Illustrated Workout 1 Exercises

Press ups

Leg raises

Illustrated Workout 2 Exercises

Pull ups and body rows

Squats

Sample Programs

Beginners program

Intermediate program

Advanced program

Your training log

Introduction

This is a twelve week program designed to get you into great shape in a short period of time. Twelve weeks may seem like a long time to some people but really, when you think about it, three months from the rest of your life isn´t really much time at all, in fact it´s about the minimum amount of time anyone with serious goals should be investing in their bodies.

Getting into shape for most people isn´t just about performing various exercises for prescribed sets and repetitions, it´s not as easy as that, it normally means lifestyle changes such as diet and general attitudes towards physical activity. It is not impossible to transform your body and your life it just takes a little guidance, some self-discipline and lots of determination, you have to want to do it, if you do it half-heartedly then you should only expect mediocre results but if you give it your all then you can expect great results, this book will help you achieve those great results and ultimately a better physique and a healthier, happier, fitter life for the rest of your life.

The course is designed around bodyweight training and exercises that you can do at home without the need for expensive gym memberships or expensive pieces of equipment. This means you can focus more of your attention on training and getting into shape without worrying about the tedious journey to and from the gym, and without having to wait for your particular piece of equipment to become free, you can just get down and train, there are no obstacles. Training in this way, a convenient, hassle free way, means you are far more likely to complete your workouts and achieve your goals. Bodyweight training also has the advantage of making you more athletic, more agile and gives you more control over your own body, it is also much easier on your joints and tendons than training with external weights, which means it´s healthier in the long run.

To complete some of the exercises in this course you will need access to something you can hang from, a pull up bar or similar would be the most obvious but anything you can get under and hang from will suffice. A decent pull up bar, either one that fits permanently into a doorframe or one that can be removed and stored away after use will probably cost you less than one month's gym membership and will last you through years of continuous use. You will also need a length of rope with a knot in either end for gripping, of sufficient length to hang over your bar to just about your waist height. This can be purchased cheaply enough from any decent hardware store. Last but not least, you will need a small notepad and something to write with so you can record your progress week after week.

Basic nutrition

This is quite possibly the most important part of this book as without an adequate diet to support your exercise routine you are already fighting a losing battle and please don´t think that by exercising you should be able to eat what you want, it doesn´t work like that. Exercise is not the magic bullet for fat loss, it is a method which should be used in conjunction with a good diet and an active lifestyle. In fact you would need to run about twenty minutes just to burn the calories off from a couple of biscuits.

The first thing most people need to change to achieve their fitness and weight loss goals is their diet, and, believe it or not, fat is not the biggest enemy that most dieters need to fear, in fact, some fat in the diet is better than none at all. The biggest enemy in the modern diet is sugar in all its forms, but more specifically, high fructose corn syrup. These days, most food companies add high fructose corn syrup to the majority of processed foods, it can be found in such things as bread, soft drinks, sauces such as ketchup and cereals to name only a few. In fact it is in almost every processed food you can think of. If you cannot find high fructose corn syrup on the ingredients list of your foods don´t be fooled by the word sugar, which is sucrose or standard white table sugar and consists of one glucose molecule attached to a fructose molecule, i.e. it´s 50% fructose.

The average American eats 141lbs of sugar per year, that's just over 10 stone.

Why do they add high fructose corn syrup to our foods? Well, because it´s cheaper and sweeter than normal sugar (sucrose), it all boils down to more profit for the big food companies.

If fructose is just a sugar then why is it so dangerous?

When we eat carbohydrates in the form of glucose, which is the preferred energy source for all living things on the planet, less than 1% of the total calories from glucose are turned into very low density lipoproteins (VLDL), in layman's terms, fat molecules.

When we eat carbohydrates in the form of fructose, which includes sucrose, 30% of those calories are converted into VLDL. This is because, fructose is metabolised in the liver differently to glucose. Glucose is converted to glycogen and is stored in the liver. Fructose is converted into VLDL (fat molecules) and is stored as fat around your arteries as well as your waist line.

So what happens when food companies remove fat from food to produce low fat meals?

Well, they replace the fat with sugar to mask the bland taste so that more of our energy intake is coming from carbohydrates and not fat, which leads to the production of more fat cells and more dangerous LDL, which can ultimately lead to obesity, heart disease, high blood pressure and type 2 diabetes.

So what can we do to avoid the curse of fructose?

Firstly, we can cut out all sugary drinks, that includes fruit juices and tea or coffee with added sugar and of course any type of soda or soft drink. We can also start to eat natural foodstuffs as nature intended, meat, vegetables, fruits, nuts, pulses and grains. This is not as bad as some people may think and it is quite easy to implement, simply buy fresh cuts of meat from the butcher and fruit and veg from the grocery store. You should aim to eat food in as close to its natural state as possible and avoid any food that has been processed or altered by man. You may have heard of this type of diet being referred to as the Palaeolithic or caveman diet.

In this type of diet safe foods that have been packaged by man are things like natural (unflavoured) yogurts, some cheeses, some pastas, rice, natural oats and nuts, everything else in a jar, tin or any type of packaging should be treated with caution and if sugar is listed on the ingredients list it should be avoided.

For more in depth information on the subject of fructose you should check out the video "Sugar: The bitter truth" which can be found at; https://www.youtube.com/watch?v=dBnniua6-oM

The last word on nutrition is - You don't need expensive supplements! If incarcerated prisoners can build strong impressive physiques on poor prison diets then this should be all the proof you need. When you consume excess protein all your body will do is convert the unused protein into energy and if those excess calories are not used then eventually they will turn into fat. Of course, all the glossy fitness magazines will tell you that you need this protein shake or that magic supplement but the truth is that most of these magazines are either owned or sponsored by the companies producing the protein powders in the first place so it is in their interests to sell them.

All you need is a healthy balanced diet (avoiding processed foods and sugar) which should consist of a good breakfast and two to three meals following throughout the day, a lot less snacking in between meals, unsweetened fluid such as water, milk, herbal teas, and, if you must, unsweetened tea or coffee. It is also advisable to eat your last meal at around 6 or 7 in the evening with maybe a herbal tea such as camomile tea before bed.

The plan

A pet hate of mine is going to any modern gym and watching the personal trainers put their clients through all sorts of fancy and frankly useless exercises which normally involve a large plastic ball or some strange embarrassing movements, you see it in all the fitness magazines as well, useless exercises that are quite frankly a waste of time. My theory for this is that the personal trainers or magazine writers are trying to prove to the poor client that they know more about fitness than their clients do so they give them some crap exercise that has never been seen before. This way the client is fooled into thinking that to get into shape he needs to come back week after week and pay more and more money to keep getting these fantastic, new exercises that no one else knows about.

My advice: **STICK TO THE BASICS!!!!!**

The basics work, they have been used for hundreds of years from ancient Greece, through gladiatorial Rome and are still being used today with every army throughout the world. How many modern armies issue their recruits with Swiss balls, TRX systems, ab rollers or any other modern gimmick to do their training? **NONE!!!!!**

That is why this plan is based around 4 basic exercises that will give you the most bang for your buck. Do not be fooled by the simplicity of the exercises, all the exercises are full compound movements which means that you can get a full body workout without having to do tons of exercises for different muscle groups.

The exercises are:

The press up or variations on the press up to work the chest, triceps, anterior deltoid and to some extent the abdominals.

Leg raises to target the abdominals, hip flexors, and thighs.

Body rows/pull ups to develop the upper back, traps, rear deltoids and arms.

Body weight squats for the whole of the legs, the butt and lower back.

Some form of cardio vascular training to get the heart and lungs working and to improve your overall fitness levels.

The 4 exercises are split into two workouts which will be done over a two week period. I have constructed a simple chart below to show you how to follow the routine.

Workout 1 WO1) – Press ups and leg raises.

Workout 2 (WO2) – Body rows/pull ups and squats.

	Week 1	Week 2
Monday	WO 1	WO 2
Tuesday	Cardio	Cardio
Wednesday	WO 2	WO 1
Thursday	Cardio	Cardio
Friday	WO 1	WO 2

As you can see, the plan is worked over a two week period giving you three workouts each of the workouts 1 and 2 interspaced with a cardio session on Tuesdays and Thursdays. Saturday and Sunday are rest days.

The cardio workouts can be a brisk walk, either in the morning or early evening for around 20 to 30 minutes, it's as easy as that. Every able bodied person can walk, can't they?

For fitter individuals you can start with a mixed jog – run session by walking between one set of lampposts and running between the next, walk, run, walk, run and so on for 20 to 30 minutes.

If you are a person with better than average fitness then a thirty minute run is a good cardio workout. Everyone from beginners upwards should be aiming to run for thirty minutes non-stop for their cardio workouts. It doesn't have to be a sprint and you're not training to do a marathon. Little by little you can improve on your workouts. You should always write down in your note book what you have done on a particular day for your training. Even if it takes you a year to be able to run non-stop it should be your goal. Time taken to achieve things doesn't really matter, after all, you're going to be doing this for the rest of your life aren't you? So, then, you have the rest of your life to improve.

When I was told by a friend and training partner that it would take the best part of a year to achieve a very strict, arm into the side, body straight, one armed press up I was a little disheartened because I thought a year was a very long time. It took me seven to eight months of continuous progressive training to get my first very strict one armed press up and looking back, that seven or eight months has been hardly noticeable in the grand scheme of things. What I want to say is that, even if it takes a year or more to achieve your goals, so what! You'll be a better, fitter, stronger person when you get there and you'll be proud of yourself for having done it.

A note on the terminology used

Throughout the descriptions of the exercises I have given targets to aim for, I have referred to these as beginners, intermediate and advanced. This is purely to describe your level at that particular exercise as the basic exercises themselves are not advanced exercises but you are at an advanced level for that exercise if you can do 40 to 50 repetitions of it.

Keep the rhythm smooth throughout your training. Using press ups as an example you should try to perform the exercise to the count of 2 to lower, a pause for 1 or 2 seconds at the bottom then a count of 2 to rise.

Body rows will be a count of 2 to raise, a pause and then a count of 2 to lower.

The cadence is important as it keeps your muscles under tension, gravity or bouncing will only rob you of the benefits of performing the exercises with good form.

The exercises

The exercises are listed under the headings, Press Ups, Leg raises etc. you will notice that there are 4 exercises under each heading, listed in order of difficulty. Simply choose 1 exercise, depending on your current level of fitness from each set and perform the recommended number of sets and reps for that exercise. Do your exercises slowly and under control at all times. If you cannot control your movement then the exercise is too hard for you.

Do not try to rush through to the harder exercises. Spending time on the easier exercises will allow your joints and tendons enough time to adapt to the greater loads you are placing on them and will help prevent tendonitis and joint pain in the future.

Rest between sets should be no more than two to three minutes.

Workout 1 Exercises

PRESS UPS

Beginners press ups

Press ups from the knees

Normal press ups

Close hand press ups

LEG RAISES

Seated leg extensions

Bent leg raises

Straight leg raises

Hanging knee raises

Workout 2 Exercises

BODY ROWS/PULL UPS

Body rows, bent legs

Strict body rows

Assisted pull ups

Full pull ups

SQUATS

Assisted squat

Half squat

Full squat

Close feet squat

Illustrated Workout 1 Exercises

Press ups

The press up is a fantastic exercise that promotes strength throughout the entire body. Do not be fooled into thinking that the press up is just for your chest and arms, the press up is a full body exercise that gives you a lot of bang for your buck. The press up will work the chest, the front of the shoulders and the triceps and by keeping the body straight you are also working the abdominals and improving your core strength, your legs even get a piece of the action as they have to remain rigid throughout the exercise.

By doing press ups you will increase the strength in the entire upper body with the emphasis on the chest front deltoids and triceps, your core strength will also improve and you will be building functional strength throughout the body which will enhance your agility. The movement will also strengthen the joints and add density to the bones helping to reduce the risk of osteoporosis.

A note on the correct form for all the press up movements

It is important when doing press ups to ensure the elbows are kept into the side of the body and not placed out to the sides. If you imagine you are going to push a car then your natural tendency will be to have your elbows into your sides, this is about the position you should aim for when doing your press ups.

The correct elbow positioning when doing press ups.

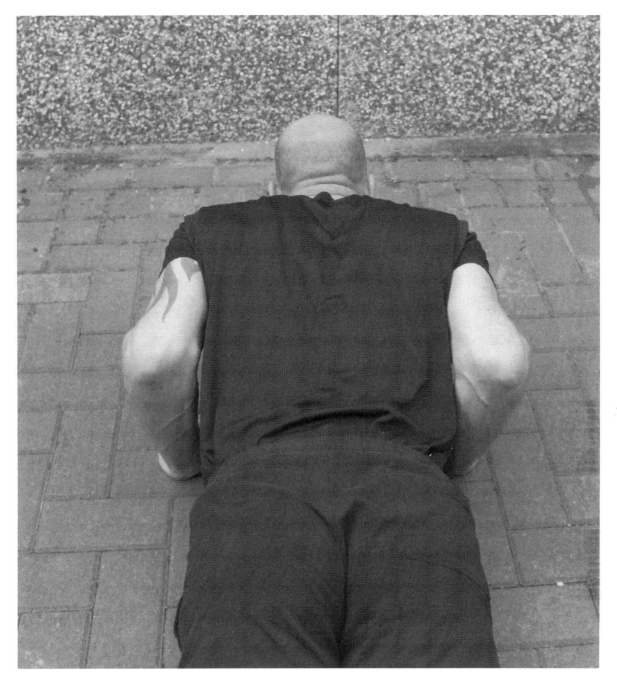

This position is the most natural and safest pushing position and will place greater stress on the triceps. The elbows out to the side position (as in the traditional bench press) will make the exercise easier but will place stress on the small rotator cuff muscles in the shoulder and could eventually lead to problems.

If you ask most body builders who do a lot of bench pressing with the elbows out to the side you will find most of them will have or have had shoulder problems. This is due to the unnatural pushing position they use to lift heavier and heavier weights.

BEGINNERS PRESS UPS

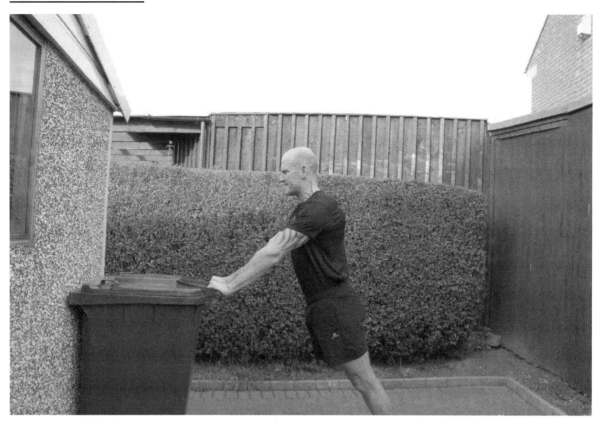

Find an object that is about waist height and stand about ¾ to 1 metre away from it and allow yourself to fall forward so that your straight arms are supporting your body with your arms about shoulder width apart and your back straight (no bend at the waist). This is the start position.

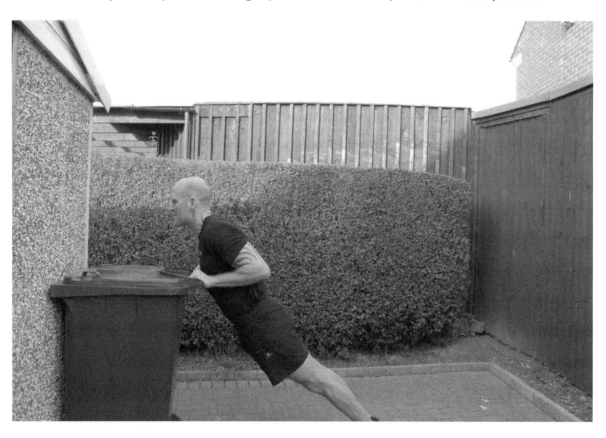

From the start position, keeping your elbows into your sides, lower yourself down under control until your chest touches the bench, pause slightly and still keeping your elbows into your sides push yourself back to the start position.

Targets

Beginners should aim for about two sets of 12 – 15 repetitions, stronger athletes should be going for around three sets of 30 repetitions and more advanced three sets of between 40- 50 repetitions.

Mark in your note book the day/date, the exercise you are doing and the amount of sets and reps you achieved. The following training session you can look back at your notes and try to add a rep or two until you reach the advanced stage. You may not be able to add reps week after week but keep training, perseverance is the key, you will eventually get there.

Try to reach the advanced stage of this exercise before moving on to the harder variations. This will give your joints and tendons time to adapt to the movements and demands you are placing on them and will benefit you in the long run.

PRESS UPS FROM THE KNEES

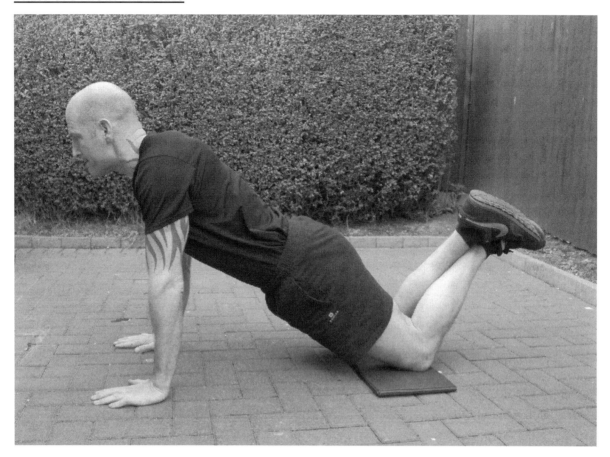

From a kneeling position place your hands on the floor about shoulder width apart, keep your back straight and your elbows locked out. This is the start position, there should be no bending at the hips, you can place your feet on the floor or have them raised as shown in the photo, whichever is most comfortable for you.

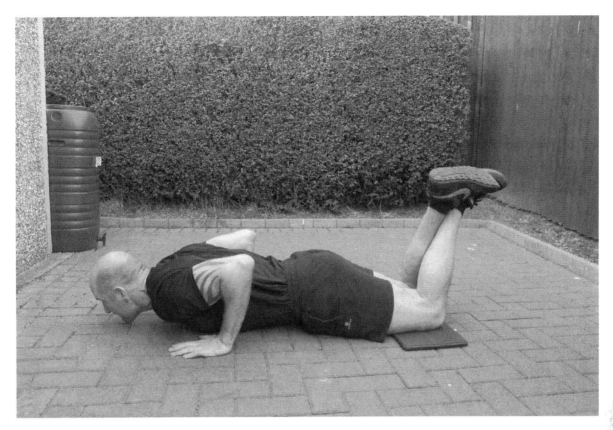

From the start position, under control, lower your chest to the floor until it gently touches the floor without taking the weight off your arms. You should not just fall to the floor and lie on it, your arms should still be supporting your weight. Pause slightly at the bottom position then push yourself back to the start position. There should be no bending at the hips at all throughout the whole movement. Keep your bum down!

The exercise should be carried out in a controlled rhythmic fashion, a count of 2 can be done in your head as you are lowering and raising your body making sure to pause slightly at the bottom to negate any bouncing.

Targets

Beginners should be aiming for around two sets of 12 – 15, stronger athletes should be going for around three sets of 20 and more advanced trainers around three sets of 30 – 40. When you can do three sets of 40 stay there for a week or two to cement your gains before moving on to the harder versions, remember, it´s not race, you have the rest of your life to improve.

I have written as a guide, three sets of 30 – 40 for example, this means you should be getting 40 for your first set, then maybe 35 for your second set and 30 for your last set or at least two nice sets of 30 for sets 2 and 3. All the repetitions should be performed with good form, no bouncing or sticking your butt up. Don´t forget to keep a record of your progress in your notebook!

NORMAL PRESS UPS

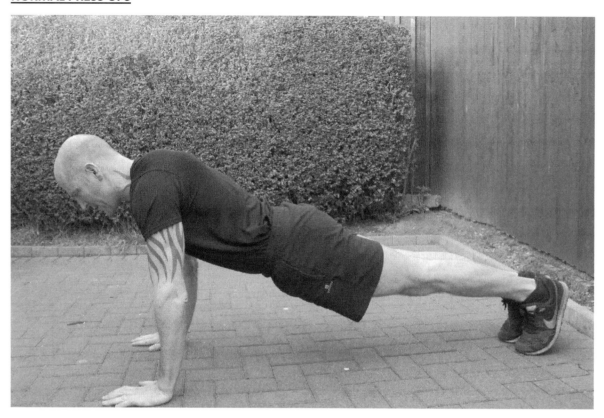

With the back straight and hands around shoulder width apart, support the body's weight on your toes and straightened arms, try to keep the legs together rather than spread apart. This is known as the front support position and is the starting point for you press ups.

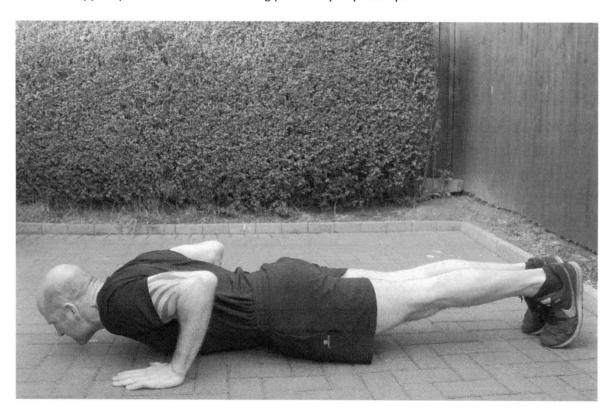

From the start position, keeping the back straight and the elbows into the side, lower the chest to the floor under control, pause briefly then push upwards back to the start position keeping the back straight throughout. A count of 2 when lowering, a pause at the bottom to avoid bounce and a count of 2 for the upward push should keep the speed of the movement about right.

Targets

If you have trained properly and reached three sets of 40 in the press ups from the knees three sets of 10 – 12 normal press ups should easily be in your reach, stronger athletes can aim for three sets of 15- 20 and more advanced athletes should be looking for around three sets of 20 – 30 good solid reps performed smoothly with a count of two on the descent a pause at the bottom and a count of two on the ascent.

If you can achieve three sets of 30, strict, slow press ups your becoming very strong, your chest shoulders and triceps will be solidly toned and sculpted and you´ll easily be ready to move on to the close hand work.

CLOSE HAND PRESS UPS

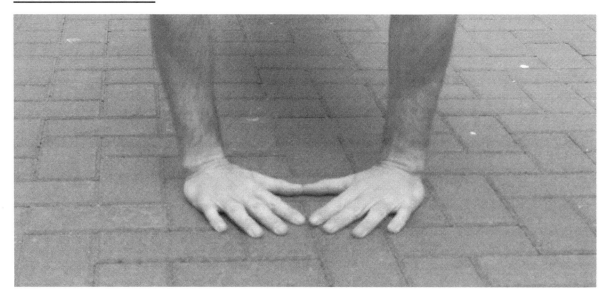

Placing the hands closer together is a big step up in the amount of strength required to perform this press up variation. The hands together position forces the triceps to take most of the load thereby strengthening and thickening the triceps muscle.

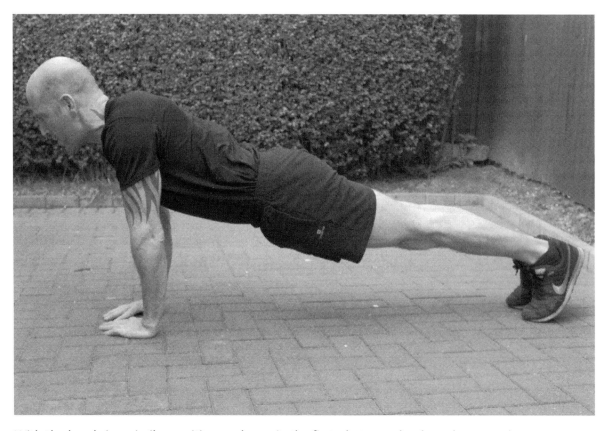

With the hands in a similar position as shown in the first photograph adopt the normal press up position with the back straight, feet together and the weight supported on the toes and hands. This is the start position.

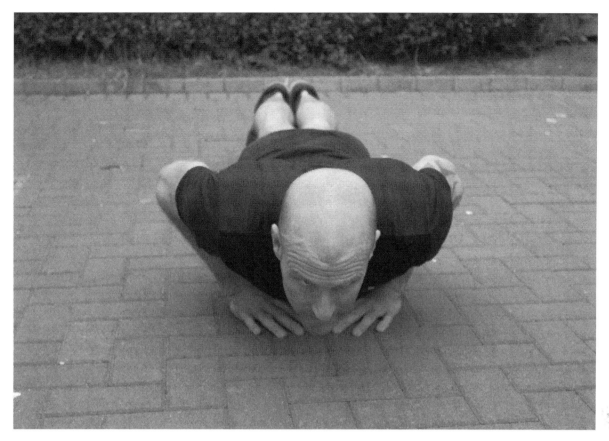

From the start position lower the chest under control until the chest lightly touches the hands, pause slightly and push upwards back to the start position. Try to keep the elbows into the sides to maintain a natural pushing position and emphasise the stress on the triceps. Remember to keep the cadence controlled by counting to 2 for the descent and again for the ascent with a pause at the bottom so there is no bouncing, you don´t want to be cheating yourself out of gains now do you?

Targets

If you have achieved the three sets of 30 normal press ups then three sets of 10 close hand press ups should not pose too much of a challenge, stronger athletes can aim for three sets of 15 and more advanced athletes should be going for three sets of around 20 – 25.

Three sets of 25 controlled, close hand press ups will have your triceps and front deltoids screaming at you. It is an excellent achievement, you should be proud of yourself. You can now begin to look at making the exercise even more challenging by simply raising the feet or adding pauses into the descent and ascent. You may even want to explore harder versions of the press up such as one handed press ups. I am planning another book which will concentrate on the more advanced exercises such as one arm press ups.

Leg raises

For a perfect midsection which is evenly developed, strong and truly functional you don´t need to do hundreds of sit ups, you don´t need to buy the latest abb cruncher gimmicky machine or go anywhere near a swiss ball. All you need to do to have a strong, powerful, functional core which will improve your agility and be aesthetically pleasing is to lift your legs. That´s right, just lift your legs and you´ll develop a stronger, better looking deeper six pack than any amount of crunches or other infomercial gimmicks could ever give you.

Modern thinking on abb work basically goes along the lines of lifting the legs works the lower abb´s and lifting the torso works the upper abb´s. this isn´t really true, the abdominal muscle is one long muscle attached at the top and bottom of its length, you can´t specify which part you want to work, any abdominal movement will work the whole muscle. Lifting the legs however, not only works the abdominals but also the hip flexors and thighs.

Raising the legs, especially when you get to the hanging work strengthens the whole waist, the hips and thighs and even the lower back. It will make you more athletic, more agile and give your core area true functional strength. Doing a crunch which so many personal trainers advocate as a way of building a six pack will only isolate the abdominals, it is not a true compound movement and will not develop the surrounding muscles of the core, the hip flexors, the lower spine or the legs, it´s about the equivalent of doing a bicep curl, a completely useless exercise for a functional body. Isolating muscles is not how the body is designed to work and has no carry over effect into everyday life. When would you ever pick something up keeping your back straight so you only use your bicep muscle? NEVER! So why train like that, it´s just not functional. The same goes for performing crunches, it´s not functional training that has any carryover to everyday life. Lifting your legs will develop stronger hips, core, spine and legs making everything you do with your legs, such as climbing stairs or getting out of a chair easier and more efficient. Plenty of carry over.

SEATED LEG EXTENSIONS

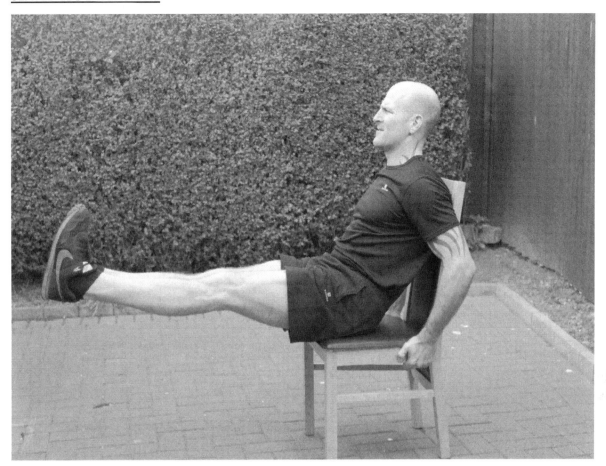

If you are new to abdominal training you may find this exercise quite challenging at first, but remember, the thing to bodyweight training is consistency, perseverance and patience. Keep training, you will get better!

Using a bench or sturdy chair sit down and from a seated position, slide your butt to the edge of the seat or bench, take a good grip on the underside to stabilise yourself and extend the legs straight out in front of you. This is the start position.

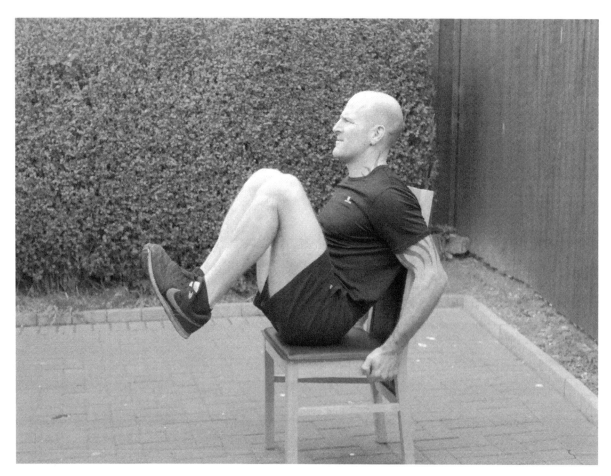

From the start position bring the knees into the chest as far as you can, pause slightly and push them back out to the start position. Keep the movement controlled at all times, it´s not about how fast you can do them it's about working your abdominals and getting the most out of every repetition you perform. As for the press ups, a count of two seconds can be used to set the rhythm, 1 & 2 in, pause, then 1 & 2 out.

Targets

Absolute beginners to this movement should aim for about two sets of around 10 – 12, intermediate trainers can aim for around three sets of 20 – 25 and advanced athletes should be going for around three sets of 30 – 40 good reps.

Build the reps up over time, remember it´s not a race you have the rest of your life. This book is about a three month plan but I´m hoping that if you complete your three months then you will continue to train and continue to improve until you become as strong and conditioned as your genetic makeup will allow.

BENT LEG RAISES

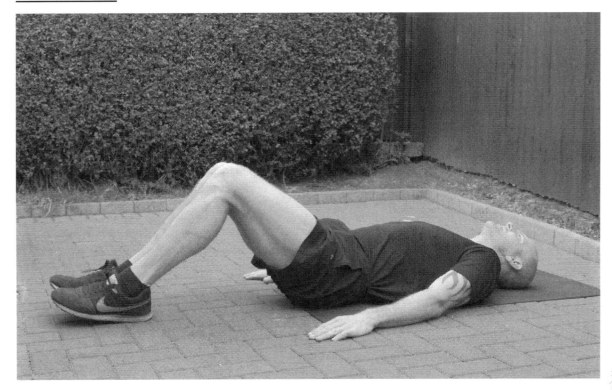

Lie on the ground with your hands slightly out to the sides and your legs bent to approximately 90 degrees. This is the start position. Do not place your hands under your butt!

It is advisable to perform this exercise on a thick carpet or to put some sort of mat under your butt to make the movement more comfortable.

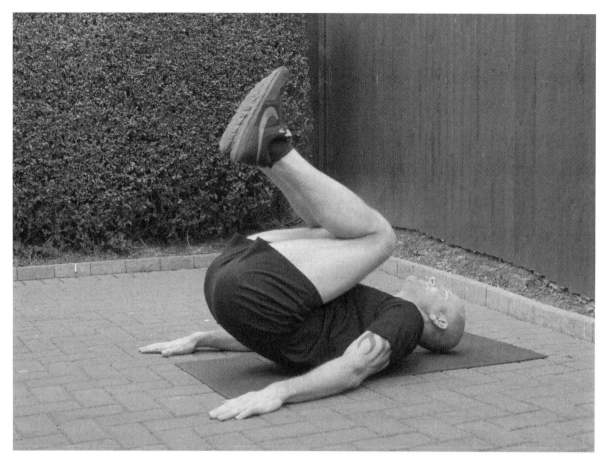

From the start position, raise the knees up to the chest maintaining the bend in the knees. Lift your hips off the floor and try to get your knees as close as possible to your chest. Lower the legs back towards the start position keeping the bend in the knees. Slightly touch the floor with the heels then go straight into the next rep, don't allow the feet to rest on the floor until you have finished your set.

Try to keep the hands out from under the butt as this makes the exercise easier, but if you are struggling with the movement it can be an acceptable starting point whilst you build up your strength to perform the exercise with your hands to the sides. More advanced athletes can take the hands out of the equation altogether by placing them lightly on the top of the head. Please do not pull on your head if you use this method.

Targets

Beginners should try to start this exercise by doing two sets of around 10 – 15 repetitions, intermediate athletes can aim for three sets of 15 – 20 and advanced practitioners should go for for three sets of 30. Be sure to reach the advanced range before moving on to more difficult leg raise variations.

ARCH HOLD

A lot of people complain about lower back pain when performing leg raises. This will subside eventually once your lower back muscles strengthen.

If you are one of these people you can introduce this hold after your leg raises. It´s very simple, just hold the position for 15 seconds, build up the time slowly until you can hold for 30 seconds. you can go for a full minute if you wish but you will probably find that after a month or so of 30 second holds that you don´t suffer lower back pain any more during your leg raises.

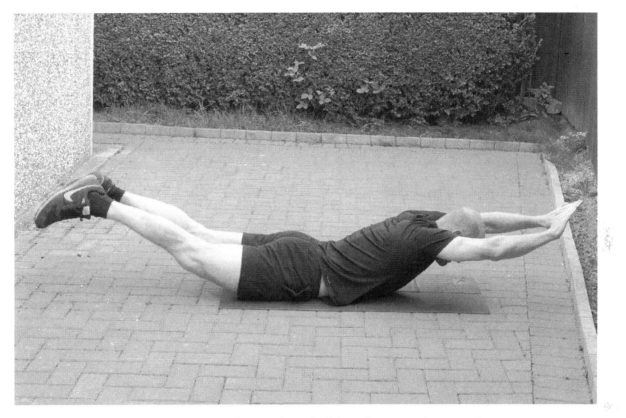

If necessary hold your arms at your sides until you build up the strength to get them out over your head.

STRAIGHT LEG RAISES

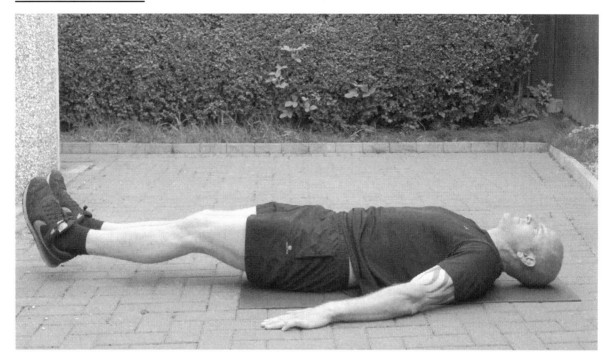

Lie on your back with your arms at the sides and your legs straight with the toes slightly pointed and your heels off the floor by a few centimetres. Do not be tempted to put your hands under your backside. This is the start position.

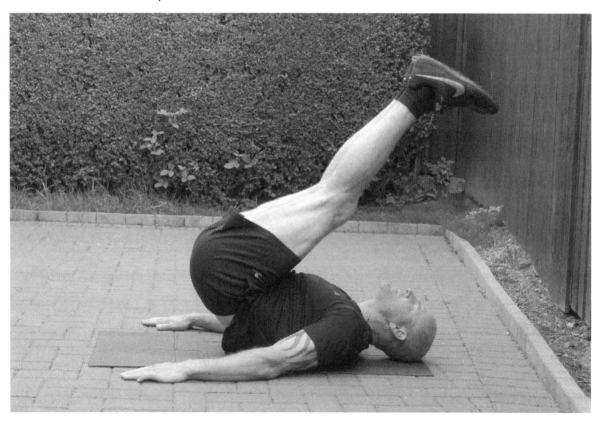

From the start position lift the legs from the ground until they are a little past the vertical then lower back down to only slightly touch the ground before beginning the next rep. Remember to keep the movement controlled throughout the whole of the exercise by giving a count of two for both the upward and lowering portions of the exercise. The feet should not rest on the floor at any point during your set but only touch it ever so slightly.

Targets

Beginners should aim for around one set of 5 – 8 repetitions. Stronger athletes can add another set and go for two sets of 10 – 15. Try to reach two sets of 20 clean, controlled reps for this exercise before moving to the hanging work.

HANGING KNEE RAISES

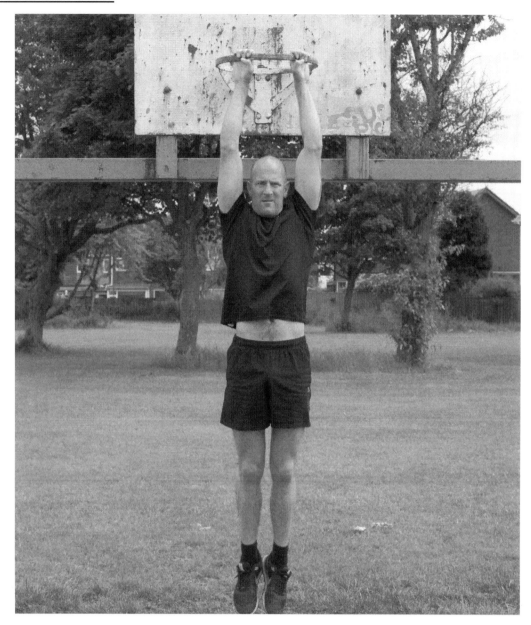

Find a suitable place to hang from where your feet are clear of the ground with your legs hanging freely down. Ensure to keep a slight kink in the elbows to protect the joint and also to pull your shoulders in slightly for the same reason. This is the start position.

To protect your joints keep a slight kink in the elbows and your shoulders tight for all hanging work. To ensure your shoulders are "tight" whilst performing this exercise simply pull them down slightly towards your back and try to bring your shoulder blades together by a quarter or so inch. This will protect the tendons from over extending and stretching.

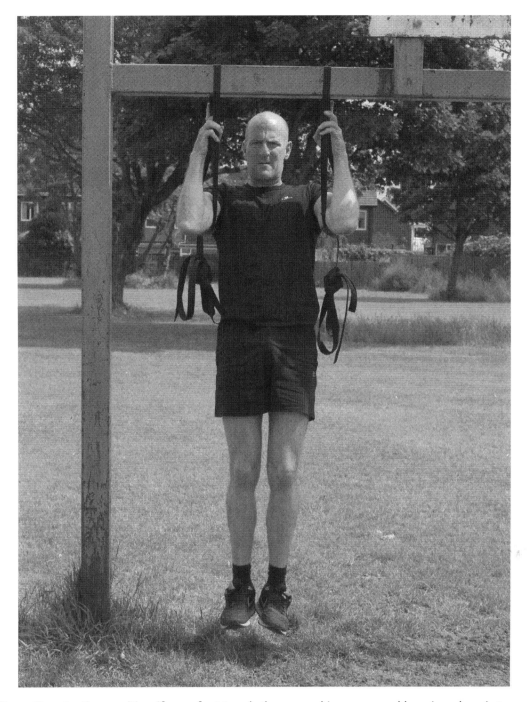

An alternative starting position if your feet touch the ground in your usual hanging place is to use two sturdy belts around your bar to support yourself under the triceps and lift the knees to the chest whilst holding yourself up. Here I have used two adjustable luggage straps.

Whichever method you use try to keep the exercise smooth and controlled and avoid swinging. Swinging will make the exercise much easier to perform but will be much less beneficial in the development of pure leg, hip and core power.

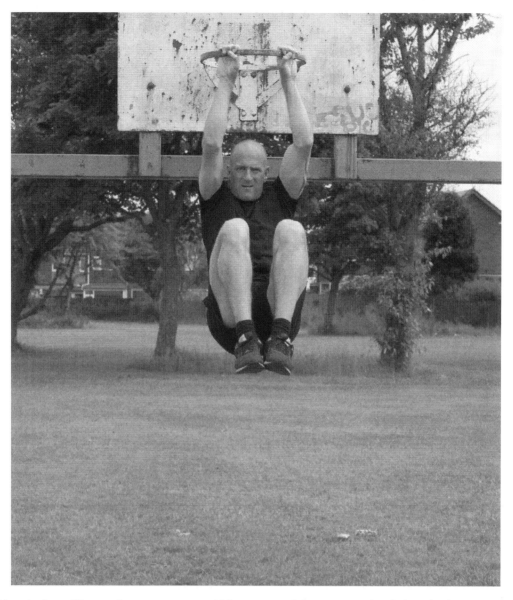

From the start position, using pure core and hip power without any swing bring the knees up to the chest in a controlled fashion. Pause slightly at the top of the movement before allowing them to straighten out under control. Do not allow gravity to bring your legs to the straight position as this will rob you of half of the exercise and also cause you to swing which will make the exercise less efficient and easier.

The deliberate movements under control will keep the muscles under tension throughout the whole movement benefiting you in developing a super strong core and rock solid abdominal muscles. If you can trim the fat from your waistline through a sensible diet then this exercise is a guaranteed route to a six pack.

Targets

Hanging work is demanding not only for your mid-section but also for your grip and arms therefore it is essential you have achieved a good foundation in the pull up exercises and also that your abdominals and hips can cope with the movement. You can build this foundation by putting your time in on the easier exercises and I would not recommend hanging abdominal work to anyone who could not perform 20 strict straight leg raises.

If you are new to this exercise I would recommend a target of around one set of 5. More seasoned trainees can go for around two sets of 12 – 15 and advanced practitioners can aim for two sets of 20. Remember to control the movements and avoid swinging. If you are swinging up into the raises and allowing gravity to bring your legs back down then you should stay at the beginner's level until your form is perfect and continue with the straight leg raises. For example, one set of 5 knee raises followed by one or two sets of 20 straight leg raises.

Illustrated Workout 2 Exercises

Pull ups and body rows

As well as the press up the pull up is a phenomenal upper body strength building exercise that promotes strength gains in not only the large muscles of the back but also the arms and rear deltoids get a damn good workout too. Sadly the pull up is often neglected by trainee's because it is difficult to perform and is usually replaced with heavy barbell rows which place a great deal of stress on the lower back or machine work which simply doesn't deliver the same results. Be safe and strong and get pulling that body upwards! The pull up is also an excellent exercise that promotes upper body agility like no other, I mean what other exercise involves moving the whole of the body upwards. Many people will have great difficulty in performing a full, clean pull up and should therefore start with a pulling exercise which doesn't require moving the whole body, such as body rows, sometimes called inverted rows.

The body row is pretty much the opposite of a press up but instead of pushing you are pulling, it is a great way to build up to full pull ups. The exercise will develop your back, rear deltoids, biceps, forearms, trapezius, core and all the stabiliser muscles in between, it is a good exercise for all round shoulder health and can help iron out a slumped posture.

BODY ROWS, BENT LEGS

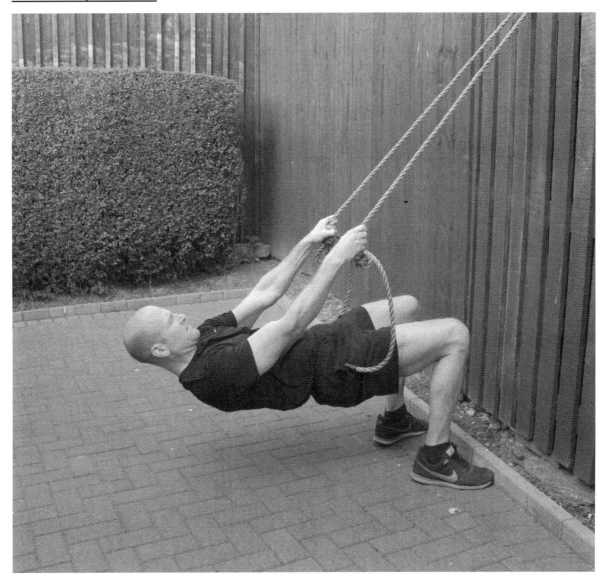

In the photo above I have slung a piece of nylon rope over the top part of a fence in my back yard, the same method works equally as well if you put the rope over your pull up station. Olympic rings which you can buy from eBay for about 20 pounds are more comfortable to grip and easier to adjust but the rope works just as well as a set of rings. Tie two knots in the rope at about waist height to help you grip it. Your back should not touch the ground when you lean back, if it does adjust your knots until it doesn't.

Grip the rope and bending at the knees lean backwards until the arms are extended. Personally, I don't like to extend my arms to the maximum and always keep a little kink in them at the bottom. That way you protect your elbows from overextending. When I say little kink, that means a little kink, not bent to a 45° angle. My elbows are slightly kinked in the photo, it's barley noticeable but my elbows are not hyperextended, that's what I mean by a "little".

With the arms extended keep the body and hips straight with the shoulders and back off the floor. This is the start position.

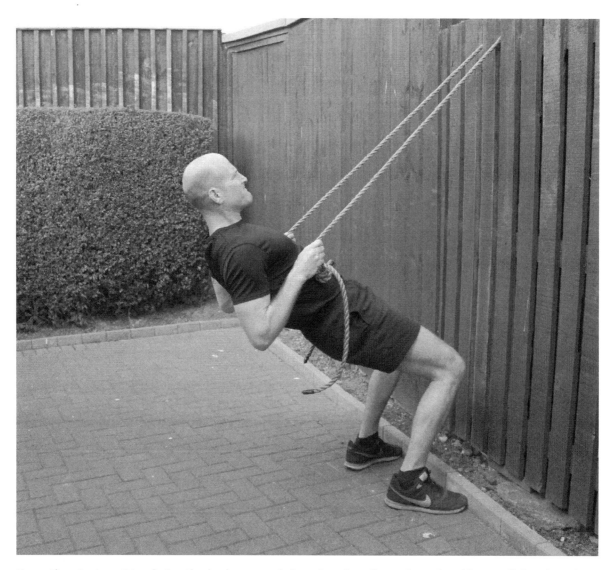

From the start position bring the body upwards keeping the elbows into the sides until the chest is level with the hands, pause slightly and then under control lower back to the start position. Maintain the tension in the torso throughout the movement and do not let the body sag. The back should be kept straight throughout, this gives the core a good isometric workout as well.

Performing this movement with the elbows slightly flared to the side and not tight to the sides will place a greater emphasis on the rear deltoids which can be a great way to rehabilitate muscular imbalances in the shoulder, a problem a lot of bodybuilders have due to too much bench pressing without any rear deltoid work. The front delts become much stronger than the rear delts through heavy pressing work. This causes them to "pull" the rear deltoids, giving a slumped, shoulders forward look and often causing pain in the shoulder region. The cure! A good dose of body rows!

If you find this exercise difficult simply heighten the rope so you are not leaning back as much and drop the body over time untill it is around parallel to the floor.

Targets

Beginers should aim for two sets of around 10 – 12 repetitions for this exercise, intermediate athletes should be looking towards three sets of 15 – 20 and the target range before moving on to harder variations of this exercise should be three sets of between 25 – 30 reps.

STRICT BODY ROWS

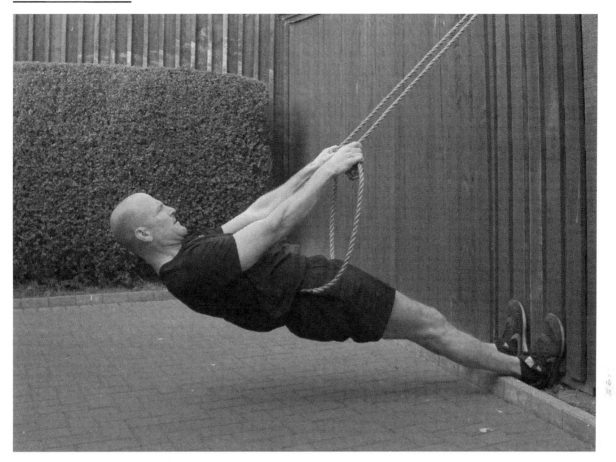

This version of the body row takes the legs out of the equation and therefore makes the exercise considerably more difficult.

Grip the rope and lean backwards, the legs and torso should be kept straight and the arms extended, this is the start position. Keep a small kink in the elbows and avoid complete extension so as not to hyperextend the elbow joint, the kink should be barely perceptible as in the photo above. Keep the body rigid throughout the movement making the arms and back muscles perform all the work required for the exercise.

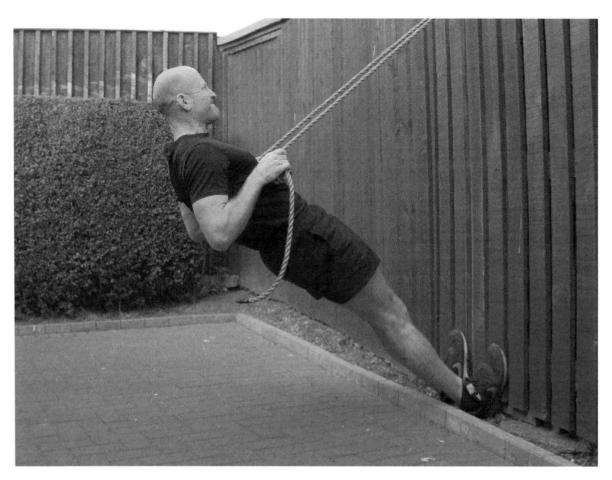

From the start position pull the torso upwards until the chest is about level with the hands. Keep the tempo controlled and pause slightly at the top before lowering under control. Pause again at the bottom before commencing the next repetition to eliminate any bounce.

Imagine you are doing this exercise on a solid bar, then the chest should be raised until it touches the imaginary bar. Try to keep the elbows into the sides unless you are deliberately trying to target the rear deltoids. The exercise can also be performed on a solid bar by the way by attaching your rope to the bar. If you would prefer to do this exercise on a solid bar why not lay a broom stick over the back of two chairs, eh voila! A solid bar.

Targets

This is a surprisingly challenging exercise to do with a strict form and good rhythm but it's definitely worth the effort and time spent building a solid foundation with rows and even to keep them in your training when you progress to full pull ups.

Beginners aim for two sets of 8 – 10 solid reps with good form and strict tempo, pausing slightly at the top and the bottom of every rep. pause at the top to recruit all the muscle fibres of the back and at the bottom to eliminate any bounce. Intermediate trainers should be doing three sets of 12 – 15 and more advanced three sets of 15 – 20.

ASSISTED PULL UPS

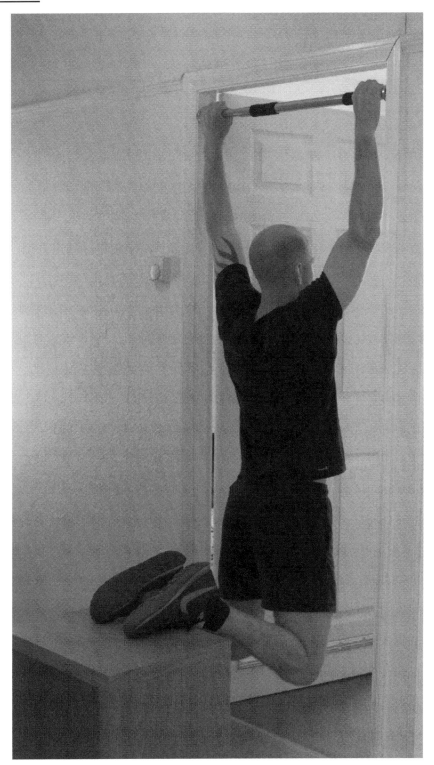

Place a chair or small platform of some sort under your pull up station and slightly to the rear. Grab the bar and then lift your feet onto the platform as shown in the photograph.

I prefer an overhand grip for pull ups but you can use whatever is more comfortable for yourself. The under hand grip, sometimes called a chin up will place slightly more emphasis on the bicep muscle and people new to this exercise may find it slightly easier as the biceps can assist more in the pulling motion. Do not lock out your elbows but keep a barley noticeable kink in them to avoid over extending your elbow joint and keep your shoulders pulled down "into your body" as described in the hanging knee raise section. This is the start position.

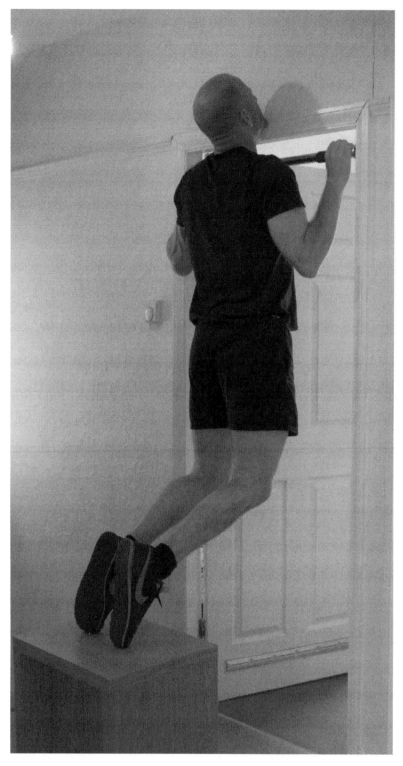

From the start position pull the body upwards until the chin is over the bar. Use the legs to assist. Try to reduce the assistance offered by the legs over time. It may also be helpful to introduce 2 – 3 negative repetitions without the chair when you become more proficient in assisted pull ups in order to develop the strength required for full pull ups.

An elastic resistance band can also be used to assist in pull ups by tying it to the bar and stretching it down to fit under the knees.

Targets

This is a difficult exercise to give a guide for as the amount of assistance you can give from the legs varies from one person to another. Your 10% will be different from my 10%. You will also find that after a few repetitions of the exercise you will start pushing more with the legs as your arms become tired. The legs resting on the chair sort of takes the weight of them out of the pull up, bear this in mind when you start pushing through them. They are on the chair to remove that weight from your pull up, it is not a leg exercise where you push most of your bodyweight upwards using your powerful thigh muscles, it is a pull exercise for your upper body pulling muscles.

If you are progressing from a good foundation of body rows then this step up should not pose too much of a problem, take it easy at first though so you can accustom your body to the movement. Try to get around two sets of 5 – 8 to start with and give minimal help from the legs. Intermediate trainers can go for around two sets 10 – 15 and the more advanced can aim for around three sets of 15 – 20.

FULL PULL UPS

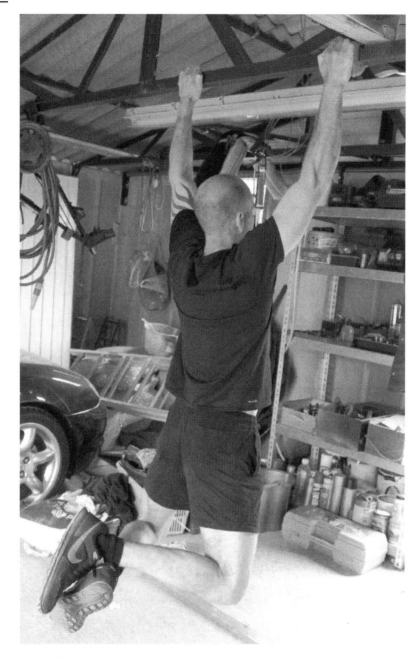

Hang from the bar in either an under hand or overhand grip depending on your preference. Here I am using the girders in the roof of the garage, you can hang from anything. Keep a barely noticeable kink in the elbows and the shoulders tight. The feet should be off the ground. This is the start position for the full pull up.

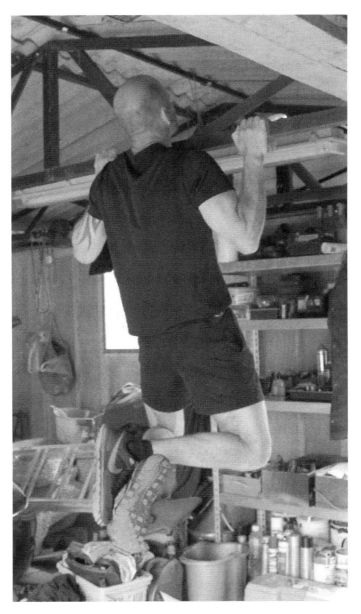

From the start position pull the body upwards until the chin is over the bar, hold slightly then return to the start position using your muscle power rather than gravity.

Kipping!!!

Kipping is when you swing and use the force of your hips and legs kicking outwards and downwards to generate momentum to push your body upwards. It´s ugly and does nothing for your strength gains, please don´t do it. You will be far better off lifting your body in a smooth controlled manner, pausing at the top for a split second then lowering under control. Your back will be screaming at you, your arms will feel like they are about to drop off, your mind will be using all of it´s cunning to get you to kip. Resist it and keep those reps smooth, your strength will improve dramatically because of it.

Pull ups are primarily a back exercise, specifically the latissimus dorsi, (your wings or lats) but normally, the day after a pull up training it is my triceps that are aching. The pull up is a strength builder for the upper back and the whole of the arms.

Targets

The pull up is a demanding exercise even for veteran strength trainers, more so if you are carrying excess weight. Leaner athletes should aim for one set of 4 – 6 heavier trainers can aim for one set of 2 clean reps.

The lucky few who don´t need to worry about dropping weight should try for three sets of around 6 – 8 and can build up to to around three sets of 10 – 12 when they are more advanced.

Normal people, mainly the ones who only need to look at a beer to gain two pounds in weight should be realistic for this demanding exercise. Two sets of 4 – 6 is good for a brawny practitioner and three sets of 8 – 10 clean, controlled reps with no kipping is very strong.

Squats

A lot of people who train regularly often neglect training their legs. This is a huge mistake as without a solid foundation of strong legs you cannot expect to achieve your full potential in any other part of your body, period!

Training legs will also help you lose weight and help to regulate your weight as they are the biggest muscles in the human body requiring lots of energy to be used when training them. Strong, well developed legs will increase your resting metabolic rate which means you will be burning more calories even when you are resting.

I have heard pretty much every excuse under the sun for why people don´t train legs, "I run" "I do cardio" "no one sees my legs" "I have bad knees" etc. etc. etc……… The real reason people don´t train legs is because it´s hard! You are using the biggest muscles in your body and squatting is a whole body exercise, yes it is demanding but it is vital if you want to reach your true athletic potential.

It´s all about mental discipline, dig deep and train those legs, you´ll be glad you did one day. And please do not go to the gym and use those mincy machines that isolate muscle groups, all they will do for you is create muscular imbalances that will only lead to problems later on. **Get squatting people!** You can´t go wrong.

Squatting down is a fundamental, functional movement that strengthens and tones the entire lower body. Introducing squats into your routine will not only strengthen the legs and tendons of the knees but also improve mobility in both the knee joint and the hips.

If you can achieve a full depth squat, ass to grass so to speak then you will have functional, agile youthful legs that will not fail you when need to move your body. Your knees and hips will have good flexibility and as you age you will retain the youthful spring in your step for much longer than other untrained, inflexible and out of shape people from the same generation.

ASSISTED SQUAT

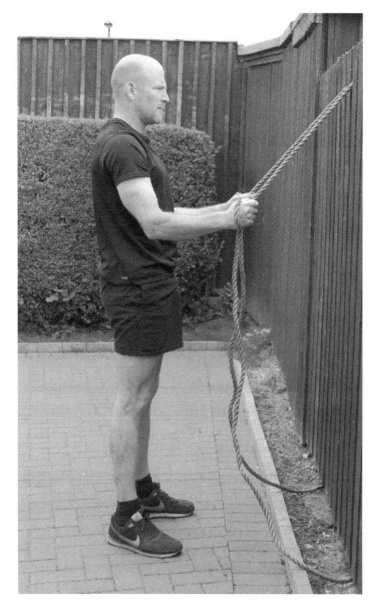

Place your rope over your pull up bar or another high anchor point and take a good grip of it at around chest height. Your feet should be around shoulder width and your toes pointing out slightly. This is the start position.

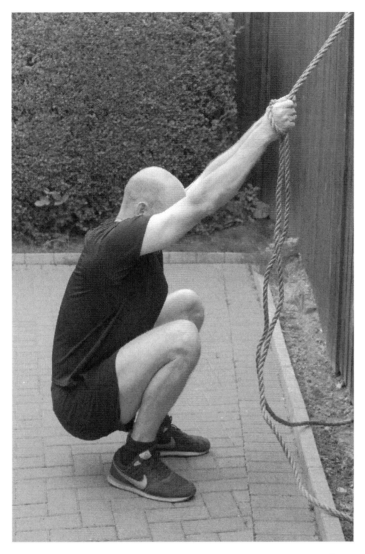

Bend your legs at the knees and lower your body (to as far as is comfortable) in a controlled fashion, using your own power rather than gravity. From the bottom position use your arms to help pull yourself up to standing again. Keep the whole movement rhythmic and controlled. Remember, a count of 2 for the descent a 1 second pause at the bottom and a count of 2 to ascend.

If you have difficulty squatting right down simply build this up over time by trying to get a low as you can with each training session.

Targets

Beginners can start with two sets of around 8 – 10 building up to three sets of 15 – 20 for intermediate practitioners. Advanced practitioners of this exercise can aim for three sets of 25 – 30.

HALF SQUAT

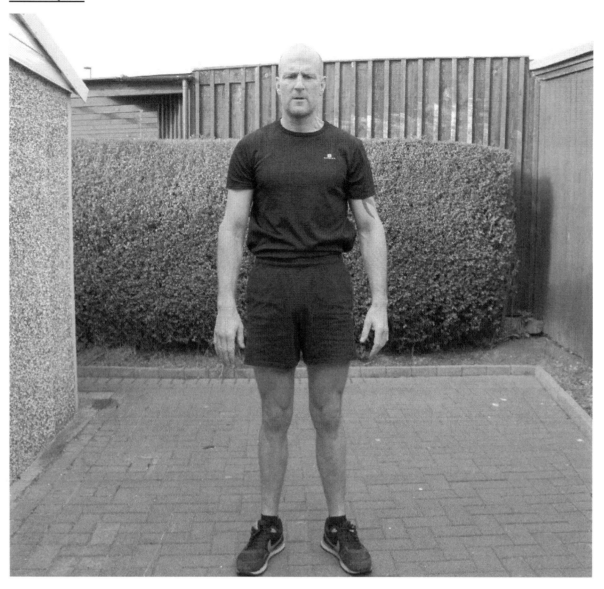

Stand in a comfortable position with the arms by the sides and the feet about shoulder width apart and facing outwards slightly. This is the start position for the body weight squat.

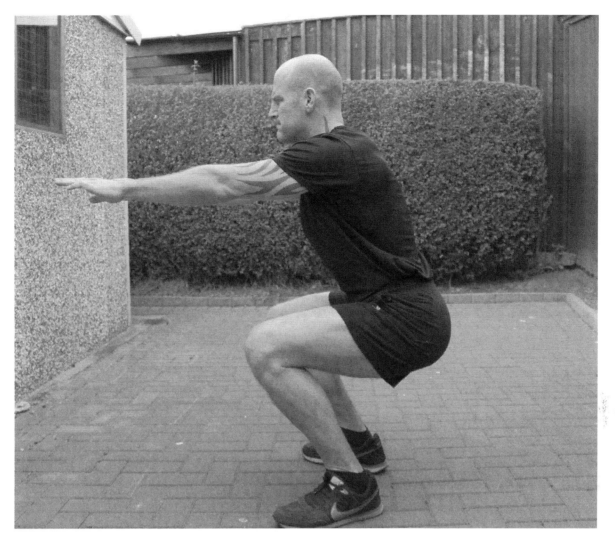

From the start position, keeping the back straight and the head up, squat down until the tops of the thighs are more or less parallel to the ground, pause slightly and return to the start position. The pause at the bottom is important to eliminate any bouncing. Do not "bounce" from the bottom of this exercise.

Bringing the arms out to the front is not an integral part of the exercise but I find it helps with the balance and also that it gives a bit of rhythm to the exercise as well as doing a little for the shoulders. It will also ensure that your back is straight as you cannot have a straight back if your arms are not parallel to the floor. You can also place the hands behind the head or across the chest if you wish but ensure the back is kept straight. Personally, I do all my bodyweight squats with my arms extended as shown in the photographs.

When performing squats keep the feet flat on the floor and do not allow the heels to rise, keep the back straight without excessive leaning forwards and angle the feet slightly. The knees should point in the direction of the feet and not bow inwards at any point. If you cannot go down to 90 degrees simply develop the depth over time and aim to eventually get to a full squat position no matter how long it takes you. By attaining a full squat position your knees and hips will be stronger, healthier and have more flexibility which will lessen the chances of further injuries.

Targets

Beginners will want to start with around two sets of 8- 10 reps building the depth and reps up to around three sets of 15 – 20 for intermediate exercisers. Advanced practitioners should aim for around three sets of 30 – 35 good solid reps before moving to harder squatting variations.

FULL SQUAT

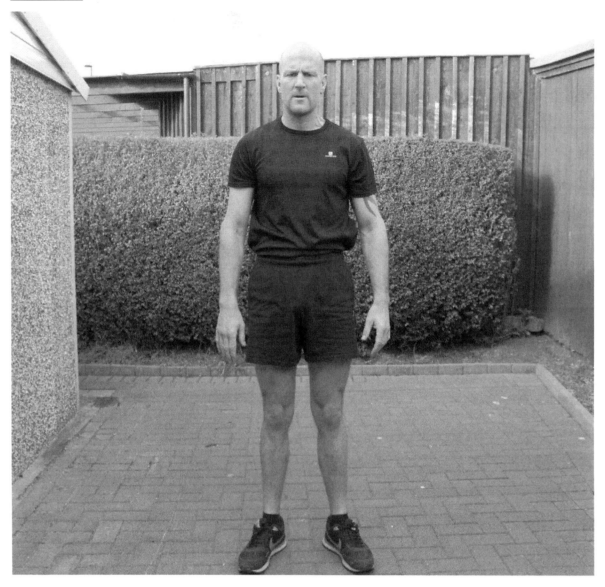

Stand in a comfortable position with the arms by the sides and the feet about shoulder width apart and facing outwards slightly. This is the start position for the body weight squat.

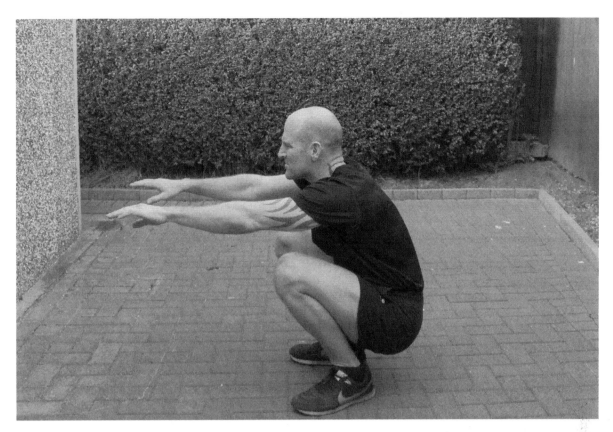

This exercise is more or less the same as the half squat only that we go as far down as we can on this one. Try to touch your calves with the back of your upper leg (your hamstrings).

From the start position lower the body down by bending at the knees. Keep the back straight as you descend without too much forward lean. Descend as far down as you can, the backs of the thighs should touch the calves. Pause at the bottom to avoid the temptation of bouncing out of the bottom portion and use pure strength to straighten the legs keeping the feet flat on the floor throughout. Keep the cadence controlled as always with a count of 2 to descend a pause and then a count of 2 on the ascend.

Targets

If you are having difficulty going all the way down keep the movements strict and controlled and simply try to add depth over time. Keep the reps to about two sets of 8 – 10 but really concentrate on getting the most from each and every rep. Intermediate athletes who have no problem performing full squats should aim for around three sets of 15 – 20 and advanced bodyweight squatters should be aiming for three solid sets of 40 reps with good cadence, plenty of control and no bouncing.

40 solid reps is challenging but keep training the movement and try to add a rep or two every few weeks and you will eventually succeed. Remember to keep a note in your training log so you can see your progress.

CLOSE FEET SQUAT

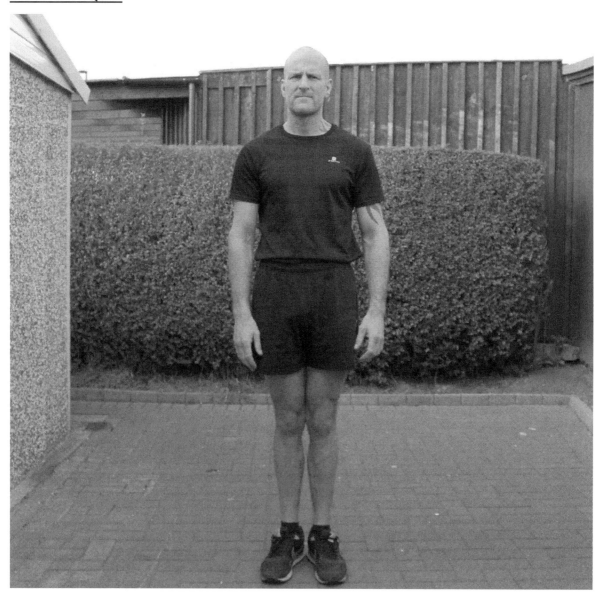

To begin this exercise adopt a comfortable standing position with the feet together at the heels and the toes facing outward slightly, the hands should drop comfortably to the sides of the body.

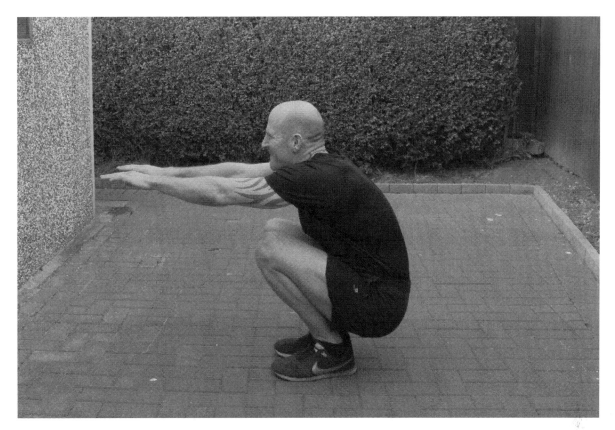

From the start position bend at the knees and lower the body down until the backs of the thighs touch the calves, pause at the bottom and then push up with the strong muscles of the legs back to the starting position.

Avoid the temptation of leaning forward to generate momentum before you push upwards. If you cannot push up cleanly from the closed feet position using pure leg power without momentum then return to the previous full squat exercise and bring the feet closer together over time.

You will probably find that you will have to bring the hands up for this squatting version to aid in the balance. You will also find that your core has to work much harder to stabilise the bottom position and stop you from falling backwards.

Targets

There is not much difference in terms of strength from full deep squats to close feet squats. The difference is with balance in the bottom portion of the exercise. If you find yourself struggling simply stick with the full squats and gradually move your feet closer together every training session.

Once you have managed to stabilise yourself in the bottom position beginners to this exercise should try two sets of 8 – 10. Intermediate athletes can go for around three sets of 20 – 25 and the more advanced can aim for three sets of 35.

Sample Programs

I am aware that a lot of people will be able to take the exercises given and construct their own programs relative their own particular strengths and weaknesses. However, there are still a lot of people out there who are completely new to training and need a structured guide to help them get started and to make exercise a part of their lives, this section is aimed mainly at the those people. I have included a beginners, an intermediate and an advanced routine which really should be used as guides rather than a set in stone routines.

Beginners program

Week 1

Welcome to the start of the rest of your life. Today you will start yourself on a journey that will benefit you for the rest of your life. Be committed and achieve your goals. The most important thing about exercises is not how many reps you can do or which advanced exercise you are on to it´s about patience and consistency. If you continue to train consistently you will reach your goals eventually but it´s not a race, be patient it will come.

Monday

2 sets of 12 beginners press ups.

2 sets of 10 seated leg extensions.

Keep the exercises nice and controlled and not too fast.

Tuesday

You may be a bit stiff after Mondays workout, this is normal if it has been some time since you last exercised, you will get used to it soon.

A thirty minute walk, find a nice park or go to the beach or somewhere pleasant and walk non-stop for thirty minutes. You can set a timer and walk out for fifteen minutes, when the alarm sounds for your fifteen minutes simply turn around and retrace your steps.

Wednesday

2 sets of 10 bent leg body rows.

2 sets of 8 assisted squats.

Remember to stay in control of your movements. Do not allow gravity to rob you of the negative portion of the exercises.

Thursday

Your legs may be feeling it a bit from yesterday but a nice 30 minute walk should help loosen them up. Your body will adjust to its new exercise regime and you won´t be as stiff the next time you train, I promise.

Friday

2 sets of 12 beginners press ups.

2 sets of 10 seated leg extensions.

Keep the exercises nice and controlled and not too fast.

Week 2

You should be feeling refreshed and ready to go again after your weekend off.

Monday

2 sets of 12 bent leg body rows.

2 sets of 10 assisted squats.

Tuesday

Your legs should be becoming accustomed to the training by now, try to push a little harder on your 30 minute walk, turning it into a brisk walk rather than a stroll.

Wednesday

2 sets of 15 beginners press ups.

2 sets of 12 seated leg extensions.

Thursday

A thirty minute brisk walk.

Friday

2 sets of 12 bent leg body rows.

2 sets of 10 assisted squats.

Week 3

Okay, we've broken you in gently for a couple of weeks to get your body accustomed to your new training program, let's start making you work now.

Monday

3 sets of 15 beginners press ups.

3 sets of 12 seated leg extensions.

Push it out for that third set. Keep good form throughout the exercises, if you lose your form simply do less reps.

Tuesday

30 minutes brisk walking.

Wednesday

3 sets of 12 bent leg body rows.

3 sets of 10 assisted squats.

Thursday

30 minutes brisk walking.

Friday

3 sets of 15 beginners press ups.

3 sets of 12 seated leg extensions.

Week 4

Another weekends rest. Are you ready for some more?

Monday

1 set of 15 followed by 2 sets of 12 bent leg body rows.

1 set of 15 followed by 2 sets of 10 assisted squats.

Try to keep your form throughout, you may find that on your third set you can't reach the number stated. Don't worry, just do the best you can but make sure you're working, no laziness here!

Tuesday

Okay, let's introduce some running into your routine. Try running between one lamp post and walking the next. If you are in an area with no lampposts set a timer on your watch or phone and run for 30 seconds walk for 1 minute.

Wednesday

1 set of 20 followed by 2 sets of 15 beginners press ups.

1 set of 20 then 2 sets of 15 Seated leg extensions.

Thursday

30 minutes of running one lamp post and walking the next or 30 seconds running 1 minute walking.

Friday

1 set of 15 followed by 2 sets of 12 bent leg body rows.

1 set of 15 followed by 2 sets of 10 assisted squats.

Week 5

Congratulations, you have completed one full month of training. I hope you haven´t missed any sessions. The first month will probably turn out to be the hardest in terms of motivating yourself, keep it up and form a habit of exercise, it will benefit you in the long run.

Monday

2 sets of 20 then 1 set of 15 beginners press ups.

2 sets of 20 then 1 set of 15 seated leg extensions.

Tuesday

30 minutes jog/walk, run 1 lamp post and walk the next.

Wednesday

2 sets of 15 then 1 set of 12 bent leg body rows.

2 sets of 15 then 1 set of 10 assisted squats.

Thursday

30 minutes jog/walk, run 1 lamp post and walk the next.

Friday

2 sets of 20 then 1 set of 15 beginners press ups.

2 sets of 20 then 1 set of 15 seated leg extensions.

Remember, you may not be able to reach the numbers given with perfect form. Give your best effort for the first set and if you need to drop a few reps for the following sets it´s okay. Do what you can just make sure you´re always working hard. If you don´t work hard you won´t improve as much as you could. No one said it was going to be easy, there's no such thing as a magic bullet.

Week 6

We'll continue to try and improve the reps this week and see if we can get three solid sets with good form. We'll keep the cardio as it is for the time being.

Monday

3 sets of 15 bent leg body rows.

3 sets of 15 assisted squats.

Tuesday

30 minutes jog/walk, run 1 lamp post and walk the next.

Wednesday

3 sets of 20 beginners press ups.

3 sets of 20 seated leg extensions.

Thursday

30 minutes jog/walk, run 1 lamp post and walk the next.

Friday

3 sets of 15 bent leg body rows.

3 sets of 15 assisted squats.

Week 7

We've built up a good routine, you should hopefully be seeing some changes to your body at this stage. Let's keep the routine the same this week and next to solidify your gains. Keep working on your form and don't go too fast on the reps, remember the 2 count down, pause, 2 count up.

Monday

3 sets of 20 beginners press ups.

3 sets of 20 seated leg extensions.

Tuesday

30 minutes jog/walk, run 1 lamp post and walk the next.

Wednesday

3 sets of 15 bent leg body rows.

3 sets of 15 assisted squats.

Thursday

30 minutes jog/walk, run 1 lamp post and walk the next.

Friday

3 sets of 20 beginners press ups.

3 sets of 20 seated leg extensions.

Week 8

We´re continuing with the same reps as before to solidify your gains.

Monday

3 sets of 15 bent leg body rows.

3 sets of 15 assisted squats.

Tuesday

30 minutes jog/walk, run 1 lamp post and walk the next.

Wednesday

3 sets of 20 beginners press ups.

3 sets of 20 seated leg extensions.

Thursday

30 minutes jog/walk, run 1 lamp post and walk the next.

Friday

3 sets of 15 bent leg body rows.

3 sets of 15 assisted squats.

Week 9

After your little consolidation period we'll now start to increase the cardio and see if we can raise our reps on the exercises.

Monday

1 set of 25 then 2 sets of 20 beginners press ups.

1 set of 25 then 2 sets of 20 leg extensions.

Tuesday

30 minutes jogging/walking. Try to run every two lamp posts now and walk one or, if you´re not using lamp posts run 1 minute walk one minute.

Wednesday

1 set of 20 then 2 sets of 15 bent leg body rows.

1 set of 20 then 2 sets of 15 assisted squats.

I know, the body rows are hard, especially when you start to get to sets of 20+ your forearms are screaming at you but dig deep, try to keep the form good and the cadence controlled. This exercise will prepare you nicely for your first full up as it builds good strength in your upper back pulling muscles.

Thursday

30 minute cardio, run two walk one lamp posts or 1 minute run 1 minute walk.

Friday

1 set of 25 then 2 sets of 20 beginners press ups.

1 set of 25 then 2 sets of 20 leg extensions.

Week 10

The number of repetitions performed are starting to become impressive. You should be developing a good base of strength by now. From here on it is simply a case of trying to increase the reps gradually. Try to add 1 or 2 reps to each exercise over your next few training sessions until you reach the advanced repetition guide for the particular exercise you are working on. When you reach the recommended advanced reps you should consider making the exercise more difficult by moving to a harder variation. Bent leg rows to straight leg or seated leg extensions to bent leg floor raises for example. Remember to record everything in your note book so you can check your progress.

Monday

1 set of 22 followed by 2 sets of maximum effort bent leg body rows.

1 set of 22 followed by 2 sets of 20 assisted squats.

Tuesday

30 minutes of cardio, running for three lamp posts and walking for one. (1min 30 seconds run, 45 seconds walk where there are no lamp posts).

Wednesday

1 set of 30 then 2 sets of maximum effort beginners press ups.

1 set of 27 then 2 sets of 20 leg extensions.

Thursday

30 minutes of cardio, running for three lamp posts and walking for one. (1min 30 seconds run, 45 seconds walk where there are no lamp posts).

Friday

1 set of 23 then 2 sets of maximum effort bent leg body rows.

1 set of 28 then a set of 22 followed by 1 set of 20 assisted squats.

Week 11

We'll continue to try and add a rep or two to our exercises always keeping good form of course.

Monday

1 set of 35 then 2 sets of maximum effort beginners press ups.

1 set of 30 then 2 sets of 25 leg extensions.

Remember to keep the reps controlled, especially on those last sets when you are tiring. If you can't keep good form then stop, you've done your maximum. Okay, you can push those last few out a bit faster, I know how it works.

Tuesday

30 minutes of cardio, running for three lamp posts and walking for one. (1min 30 seconds run, 45 seconds walk where there are no lamp posts).

Wednesday

1 set of 25 followed by 2 sets of maximum effort bent leg body rows.

1 set of 30 followed by 2 sets of 25 assisted squats.

Thursday

30 minutes of cardio, running for three lamp posts and walking for one. (1min 30 seconds run, 45 seconds walk where there are no lamp posts).

Friday

1 set of 37 then 2 sets of maximum effort beginners press ups.

1 set of 33 then 2 sets of 25 leg extensions.

Week 12

Fantastic, you´ve made it to the last week in your three month program. You will have developed a solid foundation; you can move forward from this point and start aiming for the harder exercises. Most importantly you will have developed a habit of exercise and made it a routine in your life don´t even think about stopping now. Well done to you!

Monday

1 set of 30 followed by 2 sets of maximum effort bent leg body rows.

3 sets of 30 assisted squats.

Tuesday

30 minutes of cardio, running for four lamp posts and walking for one. (2 minute run, 45 seconds walk where there are no lamp posts).

Wednesday

1 set of 40 then 2 sets of your best effort beginners press ups.

1 set of 35 then 2 sets of 25 leg extensions.

Thursday

30 minutes of cardio, running for four lamp posts and walking for one. (2 minute run, 45 seconds walk where there are no lamp posts).

Friday

1 set of 30 followed by 2 sets of maximum effort bent leg body rows.

3 sets of 30 assisted squats.

Intermediate program

I know what people are like and I know there will be people reading this who will not want to start at the beginner's level even though that is where they should start.

This program is for people who already have some training experience and have developed a decent base level of strength not only in their muscles but also in the tendons and connective tissues. I would therefore recommend that you start with the basic exercises at first even it is only for three to four weeks just to condition yourself.

Week 1

If you have gotten this far after following the beginners program, well done but you may have to start with less repetitions than given here.

Monday

3 sets of 20 press up from the knees.

3 sets of 15 bent leg raises.

Tuesday

30 minutes of cardio, running for four lamp posts and walking for one. (2 minute run, 45 seconds walk where there are no lamp posts).

Wednesday

3 sets of 15 strict body rows.

3 sets of 20 half squats.

Thursday

30 minutes of cardio, running for four lamp posts and walking for one. (2 minute run, 45 seconds walk where there are no lamp posts).

Friday

3 sets of 20 press ups from the knees.

3 sets of 15 bent leg raises.

Week 2

If you are new to exercise you will still probably feel incredibly stiff from the first week of training. Grit your teeth, you will get used to it.

We'll keep the training schedule the same this week just to get you broken in.

Monday

3 sets of 15 strict body rows.

3 sets of 20 half squats.

Tuesday

30 minutes of cardio, running for four lamp posts and walking for one. (2 minute run, 45 seconds walk where there are no lamp posts).

Wednesday

3 sets of 20 press ups from the knees.

3 sets of 15 bent leg raises.

Thursday

30 minutes of cardio, running for four lamp posts and walking for one. (2 minute run, 45 seconds walk where there are no lamp posts).

Friday

3 sets of 15 strict body rows.

3 sets of 20 half squats.

Week 3

Okay, let's start to gradually build the reps of the exercises and see if we can reach the harder variations. There is no rush, just a little improvement every week and you will get there.

This week we will also try jogging without stopping for the full 30 minutes.

Monday

1 set of 25 then 2 sets of 20 press ups from the knees.

3 sets of 20 bent leg raises.

Tuesday

3o minutes of jogging. Try not to stop just run slower if you are struggling.

Wednesday

1 set of 20 then 2 sets of 15 strict body rows.

1 set of 25 then 2 sets of 20 half squats.

Thursday

3o minutes of jogging.

Friday

2 sets of 25 then 1 sets of 20 press ups from the knees.

1 set of 25 then 2 sets of 20 bent leg raises.

Week 4

This week we are going to continue to add repetitions to the exercises in the build up to the harder variations. Keep the jogging at a comfortable pace, the most important thing is to not stop, if you´re tired just run slower but don´t walk.

Monday

2 sets of 20 then 1 set of 15 strict body rows.

2 sets of 25 then 1 set of 20 half squats.

Tuesday

30 minutes jog.

Wednesday

3 sets of 25 press ups from the knees.

2 sets of 25 then 1 set of 20 bent leg raises.

Thursday

30 minutes jog.

Friday

3 sets of 20 strict body rows.

3 sets of 20 half squats.

We will keep the body rows the same over the next few weeks to solidify your gains; it is an excellent strength builder and brilliant preparation for full pull ups. As always, keep the form and the cadence good.

Week 5

It's getting tough now eh? Those numbers are looking impressive. Keep up the hard work and make sure your form is impeccable for each exercise. I know that it becomes harder in the second and third sets, remember the numbers given in for the repetitions are a guide only. If you can't knock out 20 strict body rows on your third set, don´t worry, just work to your maximum effort. It´s the first set that is the most important.

Monday

1 set 30 then 2 sets of 25 press ups from the knees.

3 sets of 25 bent leg raises.

Tuesday

30 minute jog

Wednesday

3 sets of 20 strict body rows.

3 sets of 25 half squats.

Thursday

30 minute jog

Friday

1 set of 30 then 2 sets of 25 press ups from the knees.

3 sets of 25 bent leg raises.

Week 6

See if you can find a nice hill to include in your running route, your legs are going to love you for it.

Monday

3 sets of 20 strict body rows.

1 set of 30 then 2 sets of 25 half squats.

Tuesday

30 minute jog. Change your route to include a nice hill to run up.

Wednesday

2 sets of 30 then 1 set of 25 press ups from the knees.

1 set of 30 then 2 sets of 25 bent leg raises.

Thursday

30 minute jog, don´t forget that hill!

Friday

3 sets of 20 strict body rows.

3 sets of 25 half squats.

Week 7

We'll keep the strict body rows the same again this week, next week we'll introduce some assisted pull ups.

Monday

3 sets of 30 press ups from the knees.

2 sets of 30 then 1 set of 25 bent leg raises.

Tuesday

30 minute jog with hill.

Wednesday

3 sets of 20 strict body rows.

1 set of 30 then 2 sets of 25 half squats.

Thursday

30 minute jog with hill.

Friday

2 sets of 30 then 1 set of 25 press ups from the knees.

1 set of 30 then 2 sets of 25 bent leg raises.

Week 8

We´re moving up this week by adding assisted pull ups into our routine. You should by now have a solid foundation of body rows. Go for it!

Monday

2 sets of 8 assisted pull ups.

2 sets of 20 strict body rows.

2 sets of 30 then 1 set of 25 half squats.

I know towards the end of your sets of 8 assisted pull ups you will be using your legs more, that's ok but try not to use them too much at the beginning of your sets.

Tuesday

30 minute jog with hill.

Wednesday

3 sets of 30 press ups from the knees.

2 sets of 30 then 1 sets of 25 bent leg raises.

Thursday

30 minute jog with hill.

Friday

2 sets of 8 assisted pull ups.

2 sets of 20 strict body rows.

3 sets of 30 half squats.

Week 9

How are those assisted pull ups coming along? We'll keep those the same this week just until you get a little more used to them.

As usual we'll try to increase our numbers, squats and press ups from the knees are quite easy to improve on, you won't be able to add 5 reps a week onto your exercises when you progress to the more difficult variations, you'll be lucky if you can add 1 every few weeks on some of the harder exercises. As always, don't worry if you can't keep up, as I've said before the numbers are only a guide, every person is different and it's impossible to create a program to fit everyone. As long as you are giving it your max for every set and keeping your form good then you will improve, even if it is only 1 rep every few weeks, it's still an improvement.

Monday

1 set of 35 then 2 sets of 30 press ups from the knees.

3 sets of 30 bent leg raises.

Tuesday

30 minute jog, don't forget that hill. Try to increase your speed a little and cover more distance in your thirty minutes. In other words, start to push a little harder on your running.

Wednesday

2 sets of 8 assisted pull ups.

2 sets of 20 strict body rows.

1 set of 35 then 2 sets of 30 half squats.

Thursday

30 minute jog with hill included.

Friday

1 set of 35 then 2 sets of 30 press ups from the knees.

3 sets of 30 bent leg raises.

Week 10

We´ll keep the bent leg raises the same for a couple of weeks before introducing straight leg raises which are considerably more difficult.

Monday

2 sets of 10 assisted pull ups.

2 sets of 20 strict body rows.

2 sets of 35 then 1 sets of 30 half squats.

Tuesday

30 minute jog with hill included.

Wednesday

2 sets of 35 then 1 set of 30 press ups from the knees.

3 sets of 30 bent leg raises.

Thursday

30 minute jog with hill.

Friday

1 set of 11 then 1 set of 10 assisted pull ups.

2 sets of 20 strict body rows.

3 sets of 35 half squats.

Week 11

We´re going to keep the half squats at 35 reps now but I want you to try and increase the depth week by week until you are doing a full butt to floor squat. This may take some time to develop, depending on the flexibility of your knees, take it easy, it´s not a race, little by little every week and you will get there. The secret to body weight training is patience and consistency.

You may not get 35 reps, it depends on how much further you drop your butt. Do the best you can and always work to your maximum effort whilst maintaining good form and good rhythm.

Monday

3 sets of 35 press ups from the knees.

3 sets of 30 bent leg raises.

Tuesday

30 minute jog with hill.

Wednesday

1 set of 12 then 1 set of 10 assisted pull ups.

2 sets of 20 strict body rows.

3 sets of 35 half squats.

Thursday

30 minute jog with hill.

Friday

3 sets of 35 press ups from the knees.

3 sets of 30 bent leg raises.

Week 12

This is the final week of this program but obviously, with the gains you've made and the results you've seen with regards to your leaner, stronger body, you're not going to stop here are you? No sir! You'll continue to exercise and continue to improve, you now have all the tools you need. Now go get em!

Monday

1 set of 14 then 1 set of 10 assisted pull ups.

2 sets of 20 strict body rows.

3 sets of 35 half squats.

Go as far down as you can with the squats, it will make it harder, just do what you can, maximum effort of course, don't be lazy.

Tuesday

30 minute jog with hill.

Wednesday

1 set of 40 then 2 sets of 35 press ups from the knees.

3 sets of 30 bent leg raises.

Thursday

30 minute jog with hill.

Friday

1 set of 15 then 1 set of 10 assisted pull ups.

2 sets of 20 strict body rows.

3 sets of 35 half squats.

Advanced program

This program, with the exercises performed correctly with good form and cadence is not for the faint hearted. I would not recommend it without a solid foundation of training.

Week 1

Let´s get started then.

Monday

3 sets of 15 close hand press ups.

2 sets of 12 hanging knee raises.

Tuesday

30 minute jog. Include a decent hill in your route.

Wednesday

3 sets of 6 full pull ups.

3 sets of 20 close feet squats.

Thursday

30 minute jog with hill.

Friday

3 sets of 15 close hand press ups.

2 sets of 12 hanging knee raises.

Week 2

We'll keep the routine the same this week. If you feel you can do more then go for it but if you haven't trained for a while I would recommend taking it easy for the first couple of weeks, just until you accustom yourself to training again.

Monday

3 sets of 6 full pull ups.

3 sets of 20 close feet squats.

Tuesday

30 minute jog with hill.

Wednesday

3 sets of 15 close hand press ups.

2 sets of 12 hanging knee raises.

Thursday

30 minute jog with hill.

Friday

3 sets of 6 full pull ups.

3 sets of 20 close feet squats.

Week 3

We'll try to add a rep or two to our first sets this week. If you can't get the recommended number for the final set just give it your maximum effort.

Keep the jogging up, we're not going to change it at all throughout the whole program, it's more of a maintenance run to keep you in great shape, we're not training for marathons here.

Monday

1 set of 18 then 2 sets of 15 close hand press ups.

1 set of 15 then 1 set of 12 hanging knee raises.

Tuesday

30 minute jog, hill included.

Wednesday

1 set of 7 then 2 sets of 6 full pull ups.

1 set of 25 then 2 sets of 20 close feet squats.

Pull ups are hard, don't be surprised if you are only able to get 2 or 3 clean reps on your final set. Do your best to keep your form and cadence. Only kip if you really have to on the last rep or two. Avoid it if you can.

Thursday

30 minute jog with hill.

Friday

1 set of 18 then 2 sets of 15 close hand press ups.

1 set of 15 then 1 set of 12 hanging knee raises.

Week 4

The exercises in this routine are demanding, we'll add a rep or two every few weeks. If you feel as though you can do more then go for it.

Monday

1 set of 8 then 2 sets of 6 full pull ups.

2 sets of 25 then 1 sets of 20 close feet squats.

Tuesday

30 minute jog with hill.

Wednesday

1 set of 19 then 2 sets of 15 close hand press ups.

1 set of 15 then 1 set of 13 hanging knee raises.

Thursday

30 minute jog with hill.

Friday

1 set of 8 then 2 sets of 6 full pull ups.

2 sets of 25 then 1 sets of 20 close feet squats.

Week 5

We´ll keep the pull ups as they are this week and try to get to 20 close hand press ups by Friday. Dig deep on the squats and push those last few reps out to get to 3 sets of 25.

Monday

1 set of 19 then 2 sets of 15 close hand press ups.

1 set of 15 then 1 set of 13 hanging knee raises.

Tuesday

30 minute jog with hill.

Wednesday

1 set of 8 then 2 sets of 6 full pull ups.

3 sets of 25 close feet squats.

Thursday

30 minute jog with hill.

Friday

1 set of 20 then 2 sets of 15 close hand press ups.

1 set of 15 then 1 set of 14 hanging knee raises.

Week 6

The only thing changing this week is that we'll get to 2 sets of 15 hanging knee raises. You must have a rock hard mid-section by now, hanging knee raises are hard and they build a solid mid-section.

Monday

1 set of 8 then 2 sets of 6 full pull ups.

3 sets of 25 close feet squats.

Tuesday

30 minute jog with hill.

Wednesday

1 set of 20 then 2 sets of 15 close hand press ups.

2 sets of 15 hanging knee raises.

Thursday

30 minute jog with hill.

Friday

1 set of 8 then 2 sets of 6 full pull ups.

3 sets of 25 close feet squats.

Week 7

Let's keep the hanging leg raises at 15 this week, keep the cadence of 2 seconds up 1 second pause and 2 seconds down and no swinging.

Monday

1 set of 25 then 1 set of 20 and 1 set of 15 close hand press ups.

2 sets of 15 hanging knee raises.

Tuesday

30 minute jog with hill.

Wednesday

1 set of 8 then 2 sets of 6 full pull ups.

3 sets of 25 close feet squats.

Thursday

30 minute jog with hill.

Friday

1 set of 25, 1 of 20 and 1 of 15 close hand press ups.

2 sets of 15 hanging knee raises.

Keep the form on the press ups, try and get to 25 on the first set and do your best on the following two sets.

Week 8

We´ll try throwing in an extra pull up this week and increase our reps on hanging leg raises. Little by little folks.

Monday

1 set of 8 then 1 set of 7 followed by 1set of 6 full pull ups.

1 set of 30 then 2 sets of 25 close feet squats.

Tuesday

30 minute jog with hill.

Wednesday

1 set of 25, 1 of 20 and 1 of 16 close hand press ups.

1 set of 18 then 1 set of 15 hanging knee raises.

Thursday

30 minute jog with hill.

Friday

1 set of 8, 1 set of 7 and 1 set of 6 full pull ups.

1 set of 30 then 2 sets of 25 close feet squats.

Week 9

We'll keep the pull ups and squats the same this week, once again, if you feel you can do more go for it. Without meeting you and training with you I can't see your progress, these programs are a guide, only you know what you can do, all I say is keep good form and don't be lazy. You will progress at your own speed.

Monday

1 set of 25, 1 of 20 and 1 of 17 close hand press ups.

1 set of 18 then 1 set of 15 hanging knee raises.

Tuesday

30 minute jog with hill.

Wednesday

1 set of 8, 1 set of 7 and 1 set of 6 full pull ups.

1 set of 30 then 2 sets of 25 close feet squats.

Thursday

30 minute jog with hill.

Friday

1 set of 25, 1 of 20 and 1 of 17 close hand press ups.

1 set of 18 then 1 set of 15 hanging knee raises.

Week 10

Sometimes it can take a few weeks just to add an extra rep or two to your routines but we´ll give it a go this week, sometimes all you need is a little push.

Monday

1 set of 8, 1 set of 7 and 1 set of 6 full pull ups.

2 sets of 30 then 1 sets of 25 close feet squats.

Tuesday

30 minute jog with hill.

Wednesday

1 set of 25, 1 of 20 and 1 of 18 close hand press ups.

1 set of 19 then 1 set of 15 hanging knee raises.

Thursday

30 minute jog with hill.

Friday

1 set of 9, 1 set of 7 and 1 set of 6 full pull ups.

2 sets of 30 then 1 set of 25 close feet squats.

Week 11

At this level it is difficult to keep adding repetitions week after week so for the final couple of weeks we'll keep most of the routine as it is. We'll try to reach ten full pull ups before the end of the twelve weeks and add a rep or two to the other exercises.

Monday

1 set of 25, 1 of 20 and 1 of 18 close hand press ups.

1 set of 19 then 1 set of 15 hanging knee raises.

Tuesday

30 minute jog with hill.

Wednesday

1 set of 9, 1 set of 7 and 1 set of 6 full pull ups.

2 sets of 30 then 1 set of 26 close feet squats.

Thursday

30 minute jog with hill.

Friday

1 set of 25, 1 of 20 and 1 of 19 close hand press ups.

1 set of 20 then 1 set of 15 hanging knee raises.

Week 12

The final week with me as your guide, I thoroughly believe in you, if you have made it this far then you have a solid foundation and a strong, toned body. I'm sure you feel better for it and have no intention of stopping your training. You have the idea now, just a rep or two here and there every few weeks and you will progress. Who knows what levels of super strength you can achieve given enough time and a consistent effort from yourself. Well done man, I'm proud of you!

Monday

1 set of 9, 1 set of 7 and 1 set of 6 full pull ups.

2 sets of 30 then 1 set of 26 close feet squats.

Tuesday

30 minute jog with hill.

Wednesday

1 set of 25 then 2 sets of 20 close hand press ups.

1 set of 20 then 1 set of 17 hanging knee raises.

Thursday

30 minute jog with hill.

Friday

1 set of 10, 1 set of 7 and 1 set of 6 full pull ups.

2 sets of 30 then 1 set of 27 close feet squats.

If you have gotten this far you may want to experiment with harder variations of body weight exercises. I am planning to write a book covering some advanced body weight methods to promote incredible strength which may interest advanced practitioners of body weight training.

Your training log

I just wanted to give you a brief section on recording your progress. I find recording your progress invaluable and it should definitely be done by you. It helps you see your improvements and you can see at a glance what you did in your previous sessions. It can also inspire you to work harder, if you see that you did ten press ups last week you know that you are capable of doing ten this week, you could also think, okay, I did ten last week, this week I'm going to do eleven.

Firstly, on a new page I write the day and date and also where I am (my life can be hectic sometimes). Then I write my exercises for the day, perform them and write down after each set the number of repetitions performed, I might also add a note on how I was feeling that day.

Here is an example of how I would keep my notes.

Monday 6th July.

At home.

Full press ups. 1x30, 1x30, 1x25

Hanging knee raises 1x15, 1x 15

I can do 3x30 next time on the press ups.

Keep the knee raises the same for a few weeks.

Tuesday 7th July

At home

Stretching

30 minute run.

Wednesday 8th July

At home

Pull ups 1x 14, 1x11, 1x8

Full body weight squats 1x40, 1x40, 1x35.

Kipped a bit on the last pull up

Squats felt good

Thursday 9th July

At home

30 minute run

Hill was hard today, legs a bit stiff from yesterday.

Friday 10th July

At Home

Full press ups. 1x30, 1x30, 1x29

Hanging knee raises 1x15, 1x 15

Couldn´t manage the thirtieth rep. I´ll get it next time.

Each day would be on a separate page, even if I just write 30 minute run on the whole page. I find it easier to refer back to them when each day has a separate page.

The exercises are written in the form of 1x30 i.e. 1(set) x 30 (repetitions).

Sometimes for laziness or because I haven't recorded the set in my notebook immediately after performing it I may write Hanging Knee 2x30 instead of 1x30, 1x30.

I always look back at my previous days training to see what I did last time and to see if I can equal it or better it this time.

Thank you for purchasing this book I sincerely hope it has been helpful to you.

If you have enjoyed it and benefited from it I would be very grateful if you could leave a positive review.

Thank you

Steve Robson

Other titles from this author.

Hand Stand Press Ups – A complete training guide to achieving full range of movement hand stand press ups.

The Comprehensive Manual of Body Weight Exercises. Fitness training you can do anywhere, from beginner to advanced.

Commando Fitness for civilians and potential Royal Marines recruits.

100 bodyweight circuits for strength fitness and conditioning.

Printed in Great Britain
by Amazon